THE GOOD PRACTICE GUIDE TO
THERAPEUTIC ACTIVITIES WITH OLDER PEOPLE IN CARE SETTINGS

THE GOOD PRACTICE GUIDE TO
THERAPEUTIC ACTIVITIES WITH OLDER PEOPLE IN CARE SETTINGS

National Association for Providers of Activities for Older People

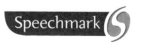

Speechmark

Speechmark Publishing Ltd
Telford Road, Bicester, Oxon OX26 4LQ, UK

First published in 2005 by
Speechmark Publishing Ltd, Telford Road, Bicester, Oxon OX26 4LQ, United Kingdom
Tel: +44 (0)1869 244 644   Fax: +44 (0)1869 320 040
www.speechmark.net

002-5214/Printed in the United Kingdom/1010

British Library Cataloguing in Publication Data

The good practice guide to therapeutic activities with older people in care settings. –
   (Speechmark Editions)
   1. Occupational therapy for the aged   2. Aged – Institutional care – Evaluation
   I. Perrin, Tessa   II. National Association for Providers of Activities for Older People
   615.8'515'0846

ISBN 0 86388 523 3

Contents

Preface

THE NATIONAL ASSOCIATION for Providers of Activities for Older People (NAPA) is a charity that was set up in 1997 to fulfil three key functions:

- To set standards of appropriate practice regarding the provision of activities for older people
- To disseminate knowledge of good practice across the network of activities providers in the UK
- To support those individuals who provide activities for older people, whether in home or care settings.

We believe that engagement in activity is essential to the maintenance of physical and psychological health and well-being. Many older people, through illness, disability or social isolation, experience diminished health and well-being as a result of disengagement from activity. This is a fact increasingly recognised by the care services, which have been shaped and re-shaped over the last two or three decades to accommodate a growing population of frail older people. As a result, carers both within and outside the professions are starting to respond; they are finding ways of ensuring that people are not disadvantaged and deprived of opportunities to engage in activity simply because they are old, or frail, or live in a continuing care setting.

However this is a relatively new area of healthcare provision and there has not, thus far, been any lead from the professions that one might expect to have an interest in this area. NAPA was established to fill the gap. It is a membership organisation, led by a multidisciplinary team of trustees who together have an extensive experience and a considerable expertise in elder care, disability and therapeutic activity. Members are from all walks of life, but are mostly activity organisers, staff from residential and day care settings and representatives of arts, disability and elder care organisations.

The key tasks set out above are addressed in three ways:

- By encouraging networking: many activity providers work in unsupported, isolated circumstances and we have found that the benefits of bringing people together for mutual support and encouragement cannot be underestimated.
- Through training: NAPA provides quality training at affordable prices, offering a range of courses concerned with the fundamental issues of using therapeutic activities in the healthcare of older people. In collaboration with City & Guilds, we have recently developed a new award – the Certificate in Providing Therapeutic Activities for Older People (see page 57).
- Through research and publication: we believe that good quality research and the dissemination of information is at the heart of progress in the healthcare field. Our research interests and our publications reflect a striving for quality and excellence in this field, alongside a need to remain earthed in the practical needs of the activity provider.

Wherever it goes, and whatever it does, NAPA is concerned about good practice in activity provision. We are delighted therefore to be able to offer the first ever good practice guide in the matter of providing activities. We trust that it will serve in a practical way to endorse our three-fold task to set a standard, to disseminate knowledge and to support the activity provider.

Tessa Perrin
Hon. Director of Training, NAPA

Acknowledgements

A PUBLICATION SUCH AS THIS is never, of course, the work of just one person. It is the product of the wisdom and experience of many and we wish sincerely to thank all those who have been a part of it – in the shaping of ideas, in the gathering of knowledge, in the constant challenge to the status quo. We are particularly indebted to those NAPA members and associates who have commented, contributed and criticised at various stages of the draft.

Tessa Perrin

CHAPTER **1**

Introduction

1.1 Why has NAPA written this good practice guide?

1.1.1 To set a standard

Within the field of activity provision for older people in healthcare settings there has never been any kind of published standard, guideline or benchmark against which activity providers can measure and evaluate their practice. As a result, what is understood (and delivered) as good practice varies greatly from practitioner to practitioner. At best this situation is unprofessional; at worst it is unethical and it should not be allowed to continue.

1.1.2 To bring together the spread of information on good practice into one publication

Information on good practice is available in the healthcare literature. It is, however, spread across a wide variety of publications, including professional journals, academic research, books and periodicals. It is difficult and time-consuming to access this information, and even more difficult and time-consuming to construct a 'whole' model of practice from the many constituent parts. This book is based on a survey of the literature and has attempted to construct that whole.

1.1.3 To disseminate knowledge of good practice

The power of the printed word is well known; it is by far the most efficient way we have of delivering a message. By means of the published book, we can reach many whom we would not be able to reach by word of mouth in training, conference or consultation. Although this means may not be ideal, in our days of severe financial constraints we can use it to reach people in a considerably more economic fashion.

1.1.4 To act as an initiative in clinical governance

There are currently in the United Kingdom no controls over the practice of activity provision in care settings for older people. There is no regulatory body for activity provision or activity providers. There is no definitive good practice guide or code of ethics. For these reasons there is also no official protection for activity providers against any accusation of malpractice. Some activity provision is carried out by occupational therapists and occupational therapy support staff and is thereby under the regulation of the College of Occupational Therapists. By far the greater part of activity provision however, is carried out by people who do not have any kind of accredited training or 'official' qualification for the task. This state of affairs cannot be allowed to continue.

NAPA has no official powers to impose any kind of regulation in this field. It does, however, have greater experience and expertise than any other collective body in the UK in matters of activity provision for older people in care settings. It therefore has an implicit authority and responsibility to take a lead in making a definitive statement on what constitutes good practice.

1.1.5 To assist care home owners/managers who wish to respond to national guidelines

Recent government initiatives have now laid upon owners/managers a statutory responsibility to provide activities for their clients. However, they offer very little in the way of guidance for the owner/manager who does not know how to fulfil this obligation. This is, in effect, specifying a destination without giving any directions as to how to get there. This book provides clear guidance for the conscientious owner/manager.

1.1.6 To offer a practice model for activity providers

This book is intended to be the activity provider's starting point, to act as a model or a guideline to signpost the activity provider in the right direction. It might also be perceived as the skeleton or basic support structure for the activity provider's core philosophy and practice. It makes no attempt to 'flesh out the bones' – there are plenty of other publications on which to draw for that purpose. In a sense, it describes a model that usually remains unspoken and therefore hidden, but without this model the practice of activity provision has no integrity and no form.

1.1.7 To make a definitive written statement of NAPA philosophy

The beliefs and standards set out in this book pre-existed NAPA's establishment as an organisation and have consistently underpinned the principles and practices of individual members of NAPA's core team over many years. It was these beliefs and standards that drew us together in the first place, but they have never before been laid down in any formal document.

1.2 What kind of a book is this good practice guide?

1.2.1 A tangible expression of NAPA philosophy

NAPA's philosophy is expressed in a range of different ways – verbal, practical and written, through training, consultation, networking and publications. This book is a crystallisation of that philosophy into a formal statement. Making such a statement is a necessary discipline, since any documented organisational 'creed' imposes a certain obligation upon its authors to abide by its assertions. It therefore acts as an integrated frame of reference for the continued good practice of NAPA.

1.2.2 A statement of best practice

This book is indeed a statement of best *practice*, though in order to define best practice it is necessary to set it in its historical and research context. Best practice is not something that NAPA (or indeed anybody else) has invented. It has evolved with a history and it draws on a large body of research evidence. Although the greater part of the book is concerned with the practice of activity provision, we would be failing in our task if we did not address the contextual development. The competent practitioner should understand the roots of the model of practice that exists within our current culture.

1.2.3 A practice model for the care setting manager and activity provider

It is our intention that managers and/or activity providers working within care settings would use this book as a framework on which to build (or improve) the practice of activity provision within their units. We would see it as a 'route map' and would use such a map to help us make an accurate assessment of where we are now, of where exactly we wish to go, and the best way of reaching that destination. Staying with this metaphor, it does not (indeed it cannot) describe the scenery along the way, the road quality or the potential for traffic jams en route, for these can only be experienced as we travel our individual journey. But we should keep it with us for reference, just in case we should get lost along the way.

1.2.4 Accessible and easy to consult

It is not our intention that this book should be read from cover to cover, but that the user should be able to turn to the required guideline quickly and easily. It is therefore set out in numbered bullet points.

1.3 How have we developed this good practice guide?

1.3.1 In line with current national trends

It is our intention that this book should be in line with current governmental legislation.

In *Care Homes for Older People: National Minimum Standards* (2000) we are delighted to find Standard 12, which states that 'The routines of daily living and activities made available are flexible and varied to suit service users' expectations, preferences and capacities'. This standard lays an obligation upon the care home to ensure that service users are 'given opportunities for stimulation through leisure and recreational activities'. Nevertheless it does leave enormous loopholes of interpretation in what exactly constitutes 'stimulation through leisure and recreational activities'. It gives no indication of best practice.

In the *National Service Framework for Older People* (2001) we applaud particularly Standard 2 on the matter of person-centred care, which we believe provides a necessary ethical underpinning to the document as a whole. Nevertheless we are sad that the indicators of supportive and palliative care outlined within this standard do not include occupation; neither do the 'domains of need' indicated as a part of the full assessment process include occupational need.

We are pleased to see within Standard 7 on mental health, a sub-section indicating that older people in residential and nursing homes and day care should be able to participate in 'a range of stimulating group or one to one activities'. This sub-section does give a short list of examples of activities.

Standard 8, the promotion of health and active life in old age, is an important section. Nevertheless it perceives health promotion primarily in the context of increasing physical activity, improving diet and nutrition and immunisation. A small sub-section does draw attention to the need for access to community leisure and learning facilities, but no other reference to promoting health through occupation is made.

Along with most other elder care organisations, we welcome these government guidelines as a significant step forward in promoting quality of care services. We look forward to the day when the relationship between occupation and health is commonly understood across healthcare professions; until then, however, it is probably unrealistic to expect any clearer directives within national standards as to best practice in this area. This guide is an attempt to make good the deficit.

1.3.2 From existing NAPA philosophy

We have drawn on the beliefs, policies and practices of the NAPA team, which are always under discussion and always open to scrutiny.

1.3.3 From a multidisciplinary expertise

This guide is not simply the product of the author, but draws on the multidisciplinary knowledge, wisdom and experience of a range of professional and lay persons. We have drawn from the occupational therapy and nursing professions, management and staff of care settings, activity providers, complementary therapists, members of elder care and disability organisations, family carers and registration and inspection units.

1.3.4 From empirical research evidence relating to occupation and health

There is an extensive healthcare literature on matters relating to occupation and health generally, and occupation in care settings for older people particularly.

CHAPTER 2

The Research

2.1 What is the connection between good practice and research?

2.1.1 Research is able to tell us exactly what constitutes good practice

All clinical and therapeutic practice in healthcare settings should be underpinned by research that is of a sufficient calibre to prove its efficacy. A drug company would not think of launching a drug into the healthcare world without subjecting it to thorough and rigorous research, often over many years. Pharmaceutical research is carried out to ensure that each new drug is safe to administer and beneficial in its effects, and in order to establish clear guidelines for the medical profession on how to administer the drug therapeutically, to whom and for what purpose. The field of therapeutic activity should not consider itself any different. Rigorous research is essential because the health and well-being of our clients is at stake.

2.1.2 Research endorses our professional credibility

The drug company that launches a drug into the public domain simply on the basis of a theory that 'it seems to work' or 'we think it works' is neither reputable nor professional in placing that public at risk. The drug company needs to know both *that* it works and *how* it works, and it can only know these things through carefully controlled empirical research.

As practitioners using activity as therapy we have similar responsibilities. If we do not know that an activity may be used therapeutically, or *why* and *how* it works, we too are placing the public at risk and we cannot consider ourselves reputable or professional either as practitioners or as organisations. Research that demonstrates therapeutic efficacy is the only legitimate foundation for practice.

2.1.3 Only evidence-based practice will survive increasing economic constraints

We live at a time when all public services are being subjected to cost-cutting procedures. Any service that has the appearance of being non-essential is vulnerable. Cuts are usually made by those who have little or no first-hand knowledge of the service(s) over which they wield the axe – politicians, civil servants and senior administrators. Therefore, unless there is empirically proven and clearly documented evidence of health benefits for what is without question a labour- and revenue-intensive therapy, we have no argument for the justification of expenditure.

2.1.4 Research is an effective defence against 'fashions' in therapy

Practice that is not earthed in empirical research is at the mercy of good ideas and fashionable theories. There is of course nothing wrong with good ideas and plausible theory; they are the seeds of creativity and development – but they must be tested. The field of elder care has seen a number of therapeutic 'fashions' come and go over recent years, with little substantial evidence of their benefits. Reality orientation, validation and, currently multi-sensory environments have all attracted enormous interest (and in some cases a considerable financial outlay) over the years, mainly because practitioners perceive them as the latest 'tool for the toolkit'. All have been good ideas; all have been built around a plausible theory; none has yet established a clear empirical support for health benefits. This is not to say these approaches do not help some people in some circumstances (there is anecdotal evidence to support this), but there is no evidence to tell us which people are helped, in what circumstances or in what way.

Doing the research ourselves, or investigating the research that others have carried out, will teach us how to handle therapeutic approaches correctly and will help us not to be swayed by fashions and trends.

2.2 What, in summary, does the research evidence tell us?
2.2.1 Changes in relation to disengagement
The research evidence tells us that the following changes are instigated when a person stops engaging in activities.

Physical changes
- Muscles atrophy and joints develop contractures
- Bone loses calcium, leading to osteoporosis and fracture
- Heart atrophies and blood pressure increases
- Risk of thrombosis and embolism increases
- Appetite diminishes
- Gastro-intestinal movement decreases and constipation increases
- Potential for urinary infection and incontinence increases
- Potential for respiratory infection increases
- Potential for pressure sores increases
- Sleep pattern is disrupted.

Psychological changes
- Decreased alertness
- Diminished concentration
- Increased irritability, impatience and hostility
- Increased tension and anxiety
- Listlessness and restlessness
- Depression and lethargy
- Feelings of oppression
- Problem-solving difficulties
- Confusion and disorientation.

All the above changes, both physical and psychological, are measurable, and indeed have been measured in the context of research projects over the last 50 years. The changes have been demonstrated in young people and old people, in healthy people and in sick people, in mentally intact people, and in people with dementia. Prolonged inactivity can, and often does, lead to physical and psychological ill health, vegetation and death.

2.2.2 Changes in relation to engagement
The evidence shows that the following changes are instigated when a person returns to activity after a period of inactivity.

Physical changes
- Muscle strength and joint mobility increases
- Bone loss diminishes and healing time of fractures reduces
- Blood pressure and potential for thrombosis and embolism diminish
- Appetite increases
- Gastro-intestinal movement increases and defaecation improves
- Continence improves

- Potential for respiratory disorders decreases
- Potential for skin breakdown decreases
- Sleep pattern improves.

Psychological changes
- Smiling, laughing and talking increases
- Initiation of, and engagement in, social interaction increase
- Alertness to environmental stimuli increases
- Concentration and memory improve
- Emotions are more readily expressed
- Agitation diminishes and relaxation increases
- Humour is manifest
- Self-assertion increases
- Self-expression is enriched
- Ability to give and receive affection increases
- Daily living function is improved.

2.3 Where can we find this research evidence?

The research evidence that supports the link between activity and health is unfortunately spread across a very broad range of periodicals and professional journals extending back some 50 years or more. For the interested reader, the essential pieces of research are listed in Appendix 2.

CHAPTER 3

The Historical Context

3.1 A changing setting for a changing clientele

Anyone who has worked in a healthcare setting over the last decade or two (or three) will have had a practical experience of the radical changes that have taken place in care settings in that time, particularly the changes in residential settings. Thirty years ago the average care home operated according to a hotel model; residents were obliged to be ambulant, continent and free of significant mental impairment. They used the home rather as a hotel – a home with meals and cleaning laid on and a certain level of support and supervision if required.

Today it is very different. People are staying alive much longer, and the population of increasingly frail, very elderly people is ever growing. Care settings have been obliged to change to accommodate this trend and the greater number now operate according to a hospital model, generally with a percentage of nursing staff.

3.2 The emerging concept of engagement

Whether or not it was society's growing awareness and change that triggered the debate on occupational need in older people is a moot point.

But this awareness can certainly be traced back to a heated debate within psychology during the 1960s, centering on what has come to be called engagement/disengagement theory. One side of the debate proposed that the norm is for people to disengage in later life from active involvement in environmental and social systems. The other side of the debate suggested that successful adjustment to late life depended upon maintaining mid-life activities and developing new ones. Both theories have been subject to much analysis and criticism, but the general view of later research in the 1970s supports the latter case. The suggestion is that a minority (probably a quarter) of people in late life are able to remain inactive and happy. This leaves a large majority whom we might suppose are not happy in inactivity. The extent to which a person's disengagement is imposed by circumstances rather than voluntarily chosen is, of course, a significant factor in the equation.

3.3 Engagement studies within psychology

This debate sparked a number of research studies relating to engagement in care settings for older people during the 1970s. These studies gave voice to a growing unease about the inactivity of older people in continuing care settings, and about the lack of opportunities available for engaging in activity. They also demonstrated the benefits of engaging people in activities.

3.4 Engagement superseded by 'therapies'

Psychology's interest in engagement appeared to wane in the late 1970s and there is little further evidence of research beyond this point. It was replaced during the 1980s by a growing interest in the remediation of functional therapies which might address the problems of old age. Reality orientation and reminiscence were introduced and rose rapidly in the therapy popularity stakes, eliciting a great deal of research but not offering conclusive evidence of therapeutic efficacy. Validation followed, though the empirical research into the effectiveness of validation has not been so prolific. All this research and development activity was taking place within psychology; there were some publications written by occupational therapists, but few of any real significance.

An observation has been made in latter years on the failure of occupational therapists to pick up and pursue the psychologists' initiatives on engagement. We might not perhaps have expected psychologists to follow through with these initiatives, for they have no professional or traditional remit in occupation. But occupational therapists have, and we have wondered if responsibility for the dilatory progress of developments in this field must rest with this profession.

3.5 The negligence of occupational therapy

Occupational therapy was experiencing a major identity crisis during the 1970s and many practitioners felt that they were losing their way as a profession. Seminal work on occupation and health in the USA during the early 1980s took the profession back to its roots and started again. A newly emerging confidence crossed the water to the UK in the late 1980s, a period that saw the first occupational therapists starting to address occupational need in continuing care settings in this country.

3.6 The rise of activity nursing

Perhaps because of the absence of a lead from occupational therapy and confusion about the role of occupational therapists in continuing care settings, nurses (primarily mental health nurses) began their own initiative in activity provision and called it 'activity nursing'. If the literature is a reflection of practice this appears in recent years to have largely died out, although there are still groups of nurses in mental health settings who consider that they have a definite remit for activity provision.

3.7 The rise of the 'activity business'

Again, very probably because of an absence of any lead from occupational therapy, the 1990s has seen the establishing of an 'activity business', which is quite separate from anything to do with occupational therapists or nurses. It is two-fold. First, the activity business has seen the creation of a new role in care settings, usually with the title of 'activity organiser' or 'activity coordinator'. Second, independent activity providers are setting up in business and selling activity services to care settings.

3.8 Government initiatives towards 'person-centredness'

Running alongside the growing awareness of the occupational needs of older people in care over the last two decades has been a series of government initiatives geared towards influencing services to recognise and treat people as individuals rather than as a homogeneous group. It began perhaps with the Wagner Report of 1988 – *A Positive Choice* – which ushered in a new era of awareness of the need of individuals for privacy, dignity, independence and choice. The initiatives continue today with the *National Minimum Standards* and the *National Service Framework*.

3.9 The reawakening of occupational therapy

The strengthening theory base of the 1980s gave rise in the 1990s to a new breed of occupational therapists who have confidence in their profession. In particular, they have confidence that their profession has something significant to offer people with a chronic disability. This has elicited a new interest in and drive towards research and development, and in the latter part of the decade, identified a broad base of evidence from empirical research for positive links between occupation and health. For the first time, occupational therapists in elder care (although sadly not the profession as a whole) are starting to take a lead in the 'activity business'.

3.10 The emergence of NAPA

1997 saw the birth of NAPA, the only organisation in the UK dedicated entirely to the promotion of therapeutic activity in care settings for older people.

3.11 A multidisciplinary, multi-agency future

The rapid growth and development of interest in and desire to collaborate with the work of NAPA is, we believe, a consequence of its multidisciplinary lead. This work is far too important and far too complex to be dominated by one profession or one agency or one group. We are, after all, not simply talking about introducing a new idea or making a statement; we are talking about changing a culture of care – the long-term care of older people. If we are going to do this, and do it well, we are going to need a multi-faceted view and an aggregated wisdom. The future lies in collaborative endeavour.

CHAPTER 4

The Changing Activity Culture

4.1 What do we mean by a 'changing activity culture'?

4.1.1 What exactly is meant by the term 'activity culture'?

This is a relatively new and unfamiliar term for most care settings, yet it is the term that best describes the changes that are taking place in this area of healthcare.

A culture might be defined as the customary beliefs, social forms and material characteristics of a social group (*Webster's Dictionary*). So we might define the term 'activity culture' as the beliefs about activity, the social forms of activity and the material characteristics of activity that are customary for a particular social group – the social group in our case being those who care for older people living in care settings.

Although we may not have used the term before, there has always been an activity culture within care settings for older people; there have always been certain beliefs and practices relating to activity and the provision of activity. It is these beliefs and practices that are changing.

4.1.2 What are the beliefs and practices of the 'old' activity culture?
These have been many and varied over the years, but four have been especially prevalent.

- The belief that older people have worked hard all their lives and do not wish to be active in old age has absolved carers from any sense of need or responsibility to provide opportunities for activity. There has therefore been no policy for, or practice of, activity provision.
- The belief that the older person, having retired from working life, is now concerned primarily with social or leisure activity has led to a policy and practice in which the provision of entertainment is understood to be sufficient to meet need.
- The belief that older people are a homogeneous group (because they are all old and frail and getting older and frailer) has led to an assumption that all enjoy and benefit from the same type of activity, and a practice that does not recognise individual need and preference.
- The belief that an activity is a group entertainment has constrained policy and practice to the exclusion of individual, self-care and work or work-like activity. This belief has also led to the notion that the activity provider should adopt the role of a Butlin's Redcoat.

4.1.3 Why are the old beliefs and practices changing?
Essentially, practice is changing because it is not meeting need. The fact that it has increasingly failed to meet need over the years has laid down a challenge to existing beliefs and caused carers to rethink and re-evaluate. There are six main reasons for change.

- The client group has changed. Thirty years ago the older person had to be ambulant, continent and mentally fit in order to reside in a care home. Admission criteria have changed as advances in community care have determined that only the most frail are now admitted to residential care.

- The politics surrounding the healthcare of older people is increasingly person-centred and related to the specific needs and wishes of the individual cared for.
- Older people themselves, and their relatives and carers, are becoming more articulate in asserting their rights in relation to service provision.
- Developing educational opportunities for healthcare practitioners is producing a more thoughtful, reflective and discerning carer who is increasingly prepared to challenge the status quo.
- Developments within the profession of occupational therapy have generated a group of professionals who are committed to taking a lead in establishing good practice in this field.
- A comprehensive research literature is now available, which clearly demonstrates the critical role of occupation in physical and psychological health.

4.2 What do we mean by 'the new activity culture'?
4.2.1 How should we define 'the new activity culture'?
The new activity culture is a culture that recognises and actively promotes the vital importance of an active lifestyle for optimum health and well-being.

4.2.2 How does the new culture understand the concept of activity?
In the new culture, an activity is understood to be any constructive (meaningful, purposeful) engagement with another person or thing. This is a concept far broader and richer than that generally embraced under the terms 'leisure', 'entertainment' or 'group activity'. This is not to disparage those activities generally included under these headings. They have their place and their benefits, but a view that understands activities only as the reminiscence group, the outing or the bingo session is a poverty-stricken view, which severely constrains good practice.

The concept of 'any constructive engagement' will not only embrace the bingo and the reminiscence, it will also include the bath, the hairdo, the table-laying, the cat-stroking, the letter-writing, the corner-shop visit for a paper and a bar of chocolate. It opens out the view, and has the potential to add a completely new dimension to practice.

4.2.3 How does the new culture understand the relation of activity to health?

The fundamental beliefs of the new culture are as follows:

- Meaningful activity is essential for maintaining physical and psychological health and well-being.
- Older people who disengage from activity through illness, disability or social isolation experience diminished health and well-being.
- Meaningful activity may be used therapeutically as an agent for positive change.

4.2.4 What impact are the fundamental beliefs of the new culture having on the practice setting?

- Practitioners of different disciplines are increasingly recognising and assuming a responsibility for providing opportunities for clients to engage in meaningful activities.
- Research evidence of positive change to health and well-being through therapeutic activity is accumulating.
- Designated personnel are being employed in the role of activity organiser/activity coordinator in order to structure and direct activity provision in the care setting.
- Opportunities for education in the matter of therapeutic activities are increasing.

4.3 How is the new activity culture evolving?

4.3.1 Is the new culture developing in all care settings across the country?

Sadly no. The rate and nature of growth varies greatly from care setting to care setting. Some units have been at the forefront of good practice for many years and some are still firmly entrenched in old cultural beliefs and practices. This is largely determined by the education and experience of the unit management team.

4.3.2 How can I develop an effective activity culture in my own care setting?

There are five key requirements for changing an activity culture in a care setting.

- An unshakeable *belief* in the potential of activity to improve a person's health and well-being.
- Demonstrable *evidence* of the capacity of occupation to improve a person's health and well-being. This may come in part from the research evidence, but the best and most convincing evidence is that of positive change in your clients as a result of the activities you have been providing.
- *Enthusiasm* for the task. Enthusiasm comes from the strength of your beliefs and is measured by the value you place on the task. It is contagious.
- A sympathetic *support and supervision* system. The above qualities will avail little without a solid support system, particularly if you are operating from a lower rung in the staff hierarchy. Positive and reliable support in the context of regular supervision will strengthen your influence.
- Ongoing *education* in matters pertaining to therapeutic activities, disability and ageing. This area of healthcare is moving very fast.

Maintaining an openness to and a grasp of new developments is a key feature of cultural change.

4.3.3 What is the key feature of an effective activity culture?

The key feature of an effective activity culture is two-fold. It operates in the context of an individual goal plan for the client, and its product is positive change in the health and/or well-being of the client. The individual goal plan is considered in detail in Chapter 5.

CHAPTER 5

The Individual Goal Plan

THE INDIVIDUAL GOAL PLAN is another relatively new and unfamiliar term, in contrast to the term 'individual care plan' which has been in use for at least two decades. It is important that we differentiate between the two. The individual care plan is, as it suggests, a plan of care and not necessarily a plan of therapy or change. It may, perhaps should, be set in the context of goals to be achieved, but this is not always the case. Essentially it sets out details of how the individual is to be cared for – routines, nursing regimes, likes/dislikes, tastes and preferences.

The individual goal plan is a plan devised in relation to the therapeutic use of activity. It should not be perceived as a completely 'other' entity, but needs to operate in concert with the care plan, and can quite conceivably be embraced within the documentation for the care plan. We use the term to emphasise that it is about therapy, about change, about moving on, about improvement. The goal plan is a dynamic, developing, constantly shifting plan, which is designed to enable clients to achieve the targets they desire, whether that is to feel happier, to walk more easily, to find a friend or simply to write a letter. The effective goal plan needs to consider and act on all the points set out below.

5.1 Gathering biographical data

5.1.1 Gathering the data

We cannot care for people effectively without a rich bank of information that defines the person who is our client. A lack of biographical information radically constrains our ability to care for our client in a person-centred way, no matter how kind, compassionate or sensitive we might be in our approach to care. The greater number of older people we meet in our care settings arrive with very little known about them. The carer has only the outward appearance to work on: the body, the disability, the behaviour. The carer usually has no idea of the person that was, the life that was, or the person that now is – submerged beneath the disability. We must have as much information as possible about the person and the life before admission so that our care is able to respond to the whole person, and not just to body, disability or behaviour.

If the person is able and willing to communicate verbally, much of the information we require can be obtained from 'the horse's mouth'. This is the best way. If the person is not able to communicate verbally for reasons of speech or language impairment or a confusional or dementing condition, we need to find the closest relatives and friends we can. We then need to gather as rich a picture as we can of every aspect of the person's life.

5.1.2 Using a data-gathering document

Efficient recording of biographical data requires a well-designed document. The well-designed document will do two things. First, it will have category headings which will guide the carer as to the subject matter required and which will ensure that all aspects are considered. A sample list of category headings can be found in Appendix 1. Second, it will be clear and easy to fill in. Time is at a premium for us all and a document must be a help rather than a hindrance.

5.1.3 Compiling a life story

A life story is, by and large, an extension, a fuller version of the biographical data collection we have alluded to above. The difference between the two is that the life story is compiled and presented as a celebration of the life rather than simply as a databank with which to inform and structure care. Considerable attention is given to presentation of the life story and carers have found very creative ways to do this. Many have used a large album (in the style of the television programme 'This is Your Life'), but life stories have also been displayed in collage and filmed on video.

We believe that some kind of a life story document should be instigated at a person's first entry into 'the system', and that it should travel with them and be added to as they pass through different care services. The potential for biographical information not to be passed on, or to 'get lost' as the person moves from service to service, is considerable, but a substantial, well-presented document should safeguard against such eventualities. It should also safeguard against the time wasted by a needless duplication of the data-gathering exercise within each new service. Preferably a document should be started when the individual is still able to make their own personal contribution.

Evidence of the benefits of life stories has shown that they are valued by family and professional carers alike. Family carers are often very moved by the attention and interest shown towards their loved one. It emphasises that their relative is valued as a person and it facilitates communication and strengthens bonds with the professionals. Professional carers value the depth of insights gained and appreciate the assistance this offers to care and goal planning. Finally, carers on both sides who use the final product in their own interactions with the person have found them to be a highly therapeutic tool, bringing pleasure and satisfaction and often dispelling distress.

5.2 Carrying out an assessment

5.2.1 Making an estimate of capacities and needs

An assessment is essentially an estimate of a person's capacities (or retained abilities) and needs and must, wherever possible, precede intervention. Assessment, like biographical data gathering, is designed to assist in informing and structuring the care plan.

5.2.2 Whose responsibility is assessment?

There may well need to be a preliminary assessment of medical condition, physical disability and/or mental state carried out by the relevant professional in order to establish baseline information. In addition, the assessment of specialist needs in relation to sensory impairment, mobility, diet etc. clearly requires the services of the professional. Thereafter, further specific assessments may be carried out by the activity provider. Our concern in this document is the assessments required by the activity provider.

5.2.3 What capacities require assessment?

We would wish to endorse the recommendations for assessment as set out in Standard 3 of the Department of Health's *National Minimum Standards* (see Appendix 3). The list of standards is, however, incomplete. We would wish to add to the list the assessment of occupational capacity and occupational need, and the assessment of emotional state (or well-being).

The activity provider uses activity as therapy for two reasons – to enable a person to do better and/or to feel better. What is needed, therefore, are assessments of doing and feeling, and we would suggest that the activity provider carries out an assessment of daily living skills and an assessment of well- and ill-being.

5.2.4 Assessing daily living skills

Most elder care settings have their own 'home-produced' format for the assessment of daily living skills. If the activity provider is comfortable with this and it elicits the information required then there is no reason to change. If there is no existing format or existing tools are inadequate, we would recommend the *Functional Performance Record* (Mulhall, forthcoming). This is a standardised instrument that covers 26 categories of daily living skill and is suitable for any client group. It can be completed by anyone who knows the client well. The information elicited by the *Functional Performance Record* will give the practitioner a comprehensive appraisal of occupational capacity. This will inform the goal plan by indicating the skill levels and skill types which an intervention needs to accommodate.

The *Functional Performance Record* is currently undergoing redevelopment. Details can be obtained from NAPA.

5.2.5 Assessing well- and ill-being

Whereas most care settings are familiar with assessing daily living skills, few are familiar with assessing well-being. The development of assessment tools for measuring well-being is a relatively new area of enquiry, but one that is increasingly seen as critical for elderly care practitioners. As yet, there is no fully standardised tool on the market, but an increasing number of practitioners are using a well-/ill-being scale originally developed by the Bradford Dementia Group (Bruce, 2000). Although designed for people with cognitive impairments, it does have a potential application for use with others who have difficulty communicating their feelings. Again, it may be completed by anyone who has spent a fair amount of time with the client.

The information elicited by the scale will give the practitioner an indication of a person's current emotional state, and suggest targets to be achieved.

5.3 Making our approach

5.3.1 A person-centred approach

Our approach to the individual goal plan should be led and structured by the client as far as possible. In the area of therapeutic activity, there is no room for prescription as a GP or physiotherapist might prescribe this remedy for that problem.

5.3.2 A negotiated approach

In the area of therapeutic activity, there is no room for experts; indeed there are no experts. The activity provider's role is that of guide and facilitator; the task is to negotiate, to work with the client as far as possible to targets of mutual satisfaction.

5.3.3 An individualised approach

Our approach must recognise our client as a unique individual with a unique set of needs, tastes and preferences. No activity is universally enjoyed and found beneficial by all older people in care settings. An activity that is highly therapeutic for Mrs Smith, may be quite counterproductive for Mrs Jones. There can be no blanket approaches in the area of therapeutic activity.

5.4 Setting aims and objectives

5.4.1 Setting the aim(s)

No *therapeutic* intervention should take place without an aim. If we are concerned with positive change, an aim will affirm what we are trying to achieve and will let us know when and whether we have achieved it or not. An aim is an end point and is established by asking (and answering) the question 'What do I want to have achieved by the end of this intervention?'. Our aims will vary according to the individual needs we are addressing, and might range from enabling Mrs Brown to walk safely to the bus stop, to ensuring that Mr Davis is less agitated and more relaxed today.

5.4.2 Setting the objectives

The objectives are simply ways of meeting aims. Once we have established an aim, we need to consider how exactly we are going to achieve that aim. So if our ultimate aim with Mrs Brown is that she should be able to walk safely to the bus stop, our objectives might be that she walks a little further each day, or with less supervision each week, until the target of the bus stop is safely reached. If our aim for Mr Davis is that he is more relaxed today than he was yesterday, our objectives might be to rearrange the environment to be less stimulating or anxiety-provoking.

5.5 Selecting the intervention

5.5.1 What activity(ies) will fulfil our objectives?

Having set aim and objectives, we need to decide upon the activity(ies) which will assist in achieving our end. So for Mrs Brown we might decide to walk with her each day, encouraging her a little further on each occasion. Or we might wheel/drive her to the bus stop and ask her to walk back as far as she can. If neither of those options are possible we might walk with her once/twice/three times around the day centre, which is the same distance as her home to the bus stop. For Mr Davis, we might rearrange the seating or the lighting, play some soft music, walk with him in the garden or use the sensory area.

5.5.2 In what context will we set these activities?

We need also to be clear about who is going to take responsibility for engaging the client in these activities and who is going to assist. Where, when and how often will they happen? These are important questions to answer, for if we take the example of Mrs Brown, frequency of walking may mean the difference between achieving or not achieving the goal. If the practice walk can only be made once a fortnight or once a week it may not be enough to make it a realistic objective. And if Mr Davis clearly responds better to some people than to others, the person who accompanies him into the garden or in the sensory area is likely to be a key feature in achieving the goal.

5.6 Getting 'fit'

5.6.1 Ensuring that client skills match activity demands

Positive change will only take place when there is a match or 'good fit' between the skills of the client and the demands of an activity. If the demands of an activity are higher than the client's levels of skill, anxiety is the result. If the demands of an activity are much below the client's levels of skill, boredom is the result. Tolerance and comfort occur when there is an equivalence between the two.

5.6.2 Adapting an activity to match a client's skills

Adapting an activity to match a client's skills essentially means that the practitioner must change one or more of three things – the task, the materials or the environment. So if we are making the *task* easier or more difficult, we might use a simpler/more complicated recipe, walk the client a shorter/longer distance, have the person do the simpler/more complex parts of the tea- or sandwich-making process. If we are making the *materials* easier or more difficult to work with, we might be using larger/smaller pieces in the mosaic, using a different texture dough/clay, making the cooking ingredients more or less obvious in terms of identification of tins and jars or location in the kitchen. If we are making the *environment* easier or more difficult to work in, we may want to increase/decrease the number of people around, have more or less noise, rearrange the furniture.

Adapting activities is sometimes simple and self-evident and many practitioners do it intuitively. So if Mrs Brown wants to improve her walking skills, most of us know without having to think too hard that she needs to walk more frequently and longer distances. And if Miss Morris is distressed by the number of people in the group to which we invite her, we know that next time we need to use a small group or one-to-one setting.

However, it is not always simple and self-evident and we are not all or always able to respond intuitively. This is particularly the case in mental health and cognitive disability, where people may be unable to tell us how they feel about their experiences. Getting 'fit' is, on the whole, a complex matter and a skill, which most of us acquire over the course of long experience. But we have to say that this is the key task of the activity provider who is using activity therapeutically; the effectiveness (or otherwise) of our interventions hinges around this.

5.6.3 Ensuring that client preferences match the selected activity

Any activity we select with or for our client must in some way be pleasurable, rewarding or satisfying. None of us will engage in an activity we see as pointless, boring or distasteful. We should apply the same principles to our client.

5.7 Evaluating the intervention

5.7.1 Why evaluate?

Every intervention using activity should be concluded with some kind of an evaluation. An evaluation is simply an estimate of the value of our intervention: that is, we need to know whether our aim has been achieved or not and why. This is a critical part of good practice for it tells us how to proceed; it is a safeguard against inappropriate and time-wasting interventions.

5.7.2 How to evaluate?

- *Ask*. Where possible, we need to discuss with our client their experiences of an intervention. This may be all that is required to let us know how to proceed.

- *Observe*. We should always be monitoring our client's non-verbal behaviours. This is particularly the case with the depressed or demented client who may well not be able to tell us how they feel or what they think. Observation is of course subjective and different individuals tend to 'see' different things. However, where we have observed large changes occurring it is not usually difficult to agree on what we have seen. So if Mrs Brown has walked twice as far today as she did yesterday, that is usually evident to all and sufficient to tell us that our intervention has been successful. Similarly, if Miss Morris has wept and left the group activity and started pacing the corridor in an agitated fashion, the evidence is irrefutable. But where changes are not so clear, or where different members of the team have different views on the outcome, we need a more formal and objective evaluation.
- *Measure*. Where changes are small or equivocal, we need to measure and the best measure is usually the one we started with at assessment. So if Mrs Brown has only taken a step or two further than she did yesterday, or if *you* think she has and *she* thinks she hasn't, we probably do need to get out the tape measure and compare the distance with yesterday's distance, or perhaps with the baseline distance we measured at the beginning of the walking plan. This is important; success is a great incentive and people need to know whether and how they are achieving. If Miss Morris's responses are not clearly obvious and she is unable to verbalise her feelings, or if your colleague and yourself have some disagreement over whether her responses are relaxation and a decrease in anxiety, or withdrawal and a deepening depression, you probably do need a formal measure of well-being. For if she is getting more depressed/anxious, this activity is clearly contraindicated.

Much of the time, asking and observing will tell us what we need to know. But if we are in doubt about the effectiveness of our intervention, we should either obtain specialist advice or discontinue it. We should never work in the dark.

5.8 Recording the intervention
5.8.1 Why is recording necessary?
We record for two reasons:

● Our team colleagues need access to what is happening to their clients in the activity setting. This is particularly the case when the regular activity provider goes off sick or on holiday and others have to take up the reins.
● We need documented proof of our interventions and their therapeutic effectiveness. We live in a day of financial constraints and professional accountability. If we cannot offer managers and/or resource providers clear evidence of our worth (that is, a record of what we do and what we achieve in terms of client health and benefits), we may well find that we are vulnerable to having posts and resources cut, or they may disappear altogether.

5.8.2 How to record
There is really no standard template that can be offered in regard to the recording of interventions and their outcomes. This will be determined in part by the nature of the interventions we are carrying out with each client, and in part by each unit's own system of documentation. As a rule of thumb, the following items of information should be recorded as a minimum:

● The nature of the intervention
● The aims and objectives of the intervention
● The date(s) of the intervention
● The outcome

- An evaluation of the outcome
- A statement of intent regarding the next intervention.

Attention to the design of recording documents usually repays the initial outlay of time. Documents need to be clear, quick and easy to complete. The reader needs at-a-glance information, which is usually best obtained from checklists, tick boxes and graphs. Documents requiring screeds of longhand are laborious both to write and to read and often result in non-compliance.

5.9 The goal plan in the overall context of care

5.9.1 The goal plan in the context of the individual care plan

The goal plan should be an integral part of the individual care plan. It is not simply the responsibility of the person designated as activity provider. All members of the staff team should be contributing to planning and setting goals in relation to therapeutic activity, whether this is in the context of staff planning meetings or simply the activity provider's liaison with the client's keyworkers.

It is wise to keep the documentation relating to therapeutic activity separate from that relating to other (non-goal orientated) matters of care (methods of handling, for example), ensuring that tastes and preferences are met. However, it still needs to be accessible to all staff. A separate section of the client's file is the best place to keep it.

5.9.2 The goal plan in the context of the unit activity programme

There is no question that thorough, person-centred goal planning is time-consuming and requires good resources and efficient organisation. In many care settings though, resourcing is such that activities are primarily carried out in the context of a weekly programme of group activities; sustained work on a one-to-one basis with clients is simply not feasible. However, this should not preclude individual goal planning. Many of the client goals we are likely to be wanting to set in relation to social interaction, engagement and well-being can effectively be embraced in the context of group activities.

If we have only the resources for a group activity programme, there will of course be many client needs we cannot address. We should not feel that we have to try and meet all needs (therein lies burnout) but we do need to prioritise according to the resources we have. Addressing one need thoroughly with a considered goal plan and intervention is good practice. Trying to address half a dozen needs in random hit or miss fashion is not.

5.9.3 Who should take responsibility in relation to goal planning?

There is clearly a case in most care settings for a designated activity coordinator (see 6.1) to take prime responsibility for undertaking goal plans in relation to therapeutic activities. This person is unlikely to run many activities him or herself, but acts as a coordinator or a liaison person between client keyworkers and staff who are running activities. It is likely to be this person who coordinates the activity programme overall, who documents the initial goal plan in collaboration with the keyworker, and who makes any significant changes to it. All staff may (indeed should) contribute to it, but the activity coordinator is the prime mover.

5.10 Risk assessment and the individual goal plan

Inevitably, if we are using activity as therapy (that is, in order to bring about positive change) we are likely on occasions to be asking the client to take risks. In our increasingly litigious society we are seeing a rapid growth in policies and practices designed to eliminate as many risks as possible from the daily life and experience of the older person in a care setting. However, life is about taking risks, whether we are boiling the kettle (potential to scald/electrocute ourselves) or crossing the road (potential to walk under a bus). When we deprive people of the opportunity to take risks, we deprive them of normal everyday life experiences.

It is usually true that safe practice is good practice; but it is not good practice if it results in a deprivation of life experience of the person concerned, or if it serves to de-skill or diminish a person's abilities. Sometimes, unsafe practice is good practice if it enriches the quality of life of the person concerned or if it enables them to improve their functional ability in a given matter.

If the activity we wish a person to engage in is likely to incur risk we need to make and record a risk assessment. We also need to evaluate and record the outcome. All care settings are required to have a risk assessment policy and practice, as well as related documentation. The practitioner should use his or her own unit's standard procedure.

5.11 Planning versus spontaneity?
5.11.1 The benefits of planning and of spontaneity
There are those who believe that planning is all-important in the matter of therapeutic activities. There are others who perceive spontaneity as more responsive to client need. The truth is somewhere in the middle and activity practitioners need to find a balance in their practice.

Planning provides a structure to practice. It acts as a discipline to practitioners who must take time to consider what they are trying to achieve across the working week and to decide a course of action. Once the plan is in place it relieves practitioners of much day-to-day and hour-to-hour decision making.

Spontaneity provides the opportunity to 'go with the flow', to respond with immediacy to the circumstances of the moment.

5.11.2 Planning and spontaneity in the context of good practice
The downside of planning is that it can act as a constraint, ignoring and stifling the positives of the present moment. The downside of spontaneity is that interventions can be too hit and miss, too random for the purposes of achieving targets. Most practitioners by virtue of their personality will

be more comfortable with one than with the other, but good practice demands a balanced approach. Spontaneity in the context of a considered plan is the order of the day.

Planning is a necessary discipline for any practitioner. Practitioners who never plan never really know what they achieve and take unnecessary risks in relation to failing to address client need. Practitioners who are never able to be spontaneous are straitjacketed and take unnecessary risks in relation to monitoring and being responsive to the immediate circumstances surrounding a client. People rarely do what we might anticipate they would do; the practitioner needs to be responsive to that. So we might then suggest that the ideal is to plan, but to be able to set aside that plan in favour of an alternative course of action should the circumstances dictate. The ability to plan and organise *and* to be flexible and adaptable are the key qualities of the activity provider.

CHAPTER 6

Resources

6.1 The designated activity provider

There are many titles and job descriptions in use across the country and across organisations for the person who undertakes the role of activity provider. Indeed there is a great deal of confusion generally about this role, about its status, about training required, about career structure and about pay. There is no regulatory body for those who hold this position and no consultative group. So in the absence of any lead from elsewhere, NAPA is attempting to fill the gap and to make some recommendations in order to set a standard for the future development of this area of healthcare for the older person.

Although we believe and are recommending in this book that it is the responsibility of all disciplines to engage their clients in activities, there is no question that at this stage of development there should be a designated person or persons within care settings who will take responsibility for ensuring good practice in the matter of therapeutic activities. This may change in time, but currently we would recommend the recognition of two distinct roles within a care setting, both having a special designation for activity provision, and both being essential to good practice.

We do realise that the creation of two posts is beyond the capacity of many care settings; indeed, the creation of one post is beyond the capacity of some. However, this book is a statement of *best* practice; it is a statement not of what currently is, but of what should be. It may be that we cannot achieve the ideal, but that is certainly what we should be reaching towards.

6.1.1 The activity therapist or activity coordinator

- *Title*. We prefer the title *therapist*, since it describes someone who is using activity therapeutically. We recognise, however, that there are some professionals who have a concern about the use of the term therapist. In deference to those concerns, we are prepared to adopt the existing title of *activity coordinator* for the time being. It remains our hope that in due course the term therapist will be debated in the wider arena and considered for adoption as the universal title for this role.
- *Role*. The activity therapist/coordinator would have a management, education and liaison role in relation to activity provision within the care setting. His or her responsibilities should be as follows:
  - to liaise with the general staff team in relation to the assessment of client need, in particular the assessment of occupational need
  - to coordinate the provision of activities in collaboration with the activity organiser/provider and other members of the staff team
  - to coordinate individual goal planning in collaboration with clients, relatives (where possible and appropriate) and clients' keyworkers
  - to coordinate efficient record-keeping in relation to individual goal planning
  - to model good practice in relation to the organising and running of activities
  - to organise training and networking opportunities for activity providers

– to establish links with, and the involvement of, local community resources

– to control the stock of equipment and materials for activity provision, and preferably the budget relating to those materials.

● *Training*. The activity therapist/coordinator should have satisfactorily completed the City & Guilds 6977 Certificate in Providing Therapeutic Activities for Older People, or an award of equivalence. Awards of equivalence should have a substantial component in how to use activity therapeutically, and a substantial component in working with the older person.

● *Status and pay*. The status of the role of activity therapist/coordinator should be equivalent to, or above that, of the role of junior management in care settings. The pay should be commensurate with that status.

● *Supervision*. The activity therapist/coordinator should receive supervision from the unit manager at least once a month. If there is an occupational therapist linked with the unit, clinical supervision from this person also would be extremely beneficial. However, it should not replace supervision from the manager, which is critical for the purposes of developing and facilitating the activity culture within the care setting.

6.1.2 The activity organiser or provider

● *Title*. We prefer the title *activity organiser*, but this does need to be understood as different from, and subordinate to, the activity therapist/coordinator.

● *Role*. The activity organiser would primarily have a provider role, with some responsibility for organising the overall unit activity programme, and for the liaison with other staff that this entails. Essentially, the role is to ensure that activities happen. The activity organiser will report to the activity coordinator, and will have the following responsibilities:

- to coordinate the unit group activity programme, ensuring that staff responsible for group activities are allocated to the appropriate shift and are aware of their responsibilities
- to provide some group activities and individual activities where possible
- to support other staff in the delivery of the activities for which they are responsible
- to contribute to the individual goal planning process
- to model good practice in relation to organising and running therapeutic activities.

● *Training*. The activity organiser is essentially a practical person who requires some organisational and group skills and confidence in the delivery of practical activities. There are many and varied training courses, available through different elder care organisations, which will equip the activity organiser with these skills. Details of organisations offering training can be found in Appendix 4.

● *Status and pay*. This role should reflect the status of a senior care assistant, and the pay should be commensurate with that position. The role is considerably more demanding than the average care assistant role, and status and pay should honour that.

● *Supervision*. Supervision for this position should be carried out by the activity coordinator, preferably once a week or once a fortnight. If there is no activity coordinator, it should be undertaken by a senior manager within the care setting. The greater the organisational responsibility required of the activity organiser, the more senior the supervision and support required.

6.2 The care staff team
6.2.1 Mutual understanding and respect for different roles
The role of the activity provider is poorly understood and poorly tolerated in many care staff teams. Two of the more common misconceptions of

care staff are that the activity provider's role is something quite separate and different from their own role; also, that it is the easy job, considerably less demanding than their own. It is the responsibility of activity providers and their supervisors to work against these prejudices, for until there is a mutual respect and a valuing of different roles, activity provision will suffer.

Essentially this is a matter of education and good communication, and activity providers and their supervisors will have to take the initiative in both areas. It rarely comes from the general staff team. New care staff must be clear about the role of the activity provider. The new activity provider must be clear about the different roles within the care staff team. All must be clear about the areas of overlap and liaison.

6.2.2 Harnessing staff skills

Most staff teams are a rich resource of skills which may be tapped for the activity programme. One can cut hair, another can play the accordion, another has just done an evening class on flower arranging. Even the staff member who will not generally participate in client activities can often be persuaded to contribute their specific skill. This approach values all participants and can often help to break down barriers between activity staff and care staff. Quite aside from that, most of us are so short of resources that it is simply folly not to use the skills that are available on the 'shop floor'.

6.3 Volunteers and relatives

6.3.1 Adopting the volunteer or relative into the activity culture

Like the staff team, volunteers and relatives can be a rich resource of talents and skills that the activity provider can put to good use. They can, however, be a mixed blessing and they need to be engaged with caution. Most volunteers volunteer (in part at least) to meet their own needs. There is nothing wrong with this in principle, provided that the volunteer's needs do not take precedence over the needs of the client.

If volunteers are draining the activity culture rather than contributing to it, they should not be accommodated.

The unit needs to have a carefully considered screening process for volunteers, particularly if they are to be drawn from a volunteer bureau rather than a known group of relatives or other associates. It is much easier not to engage a volunteer, than to 'lose' an unsuitable one. The screening process needs to establish:

- What skills you require of the volunteer
- Who is to seek the volunteer and from where
- Who is to carry out the interview/selection process
- What kind of contribution you require of the volunteer
- When and how often you require them
- Who will supervise them.

6.3.2 Managing the volunteer

It is very important that a volunteer is engaged to contribute a specific skill (such as playing the piano) or to carry out a specific task (for example, to help feed residents at lunchtime). The volunteer scenario in which a person is engaged 'to help out' or 'to assist where necessary' often fails because all parties are unclear about the person's role and what can reasonably be demanded of them. It also makes the monitoring and evaluation of their contribution difficult.

Most volunteers need clear direction, especially if they are unfamiliar with the client group. They need to know who they can receive direction from and when. They also need to know whom they are to assist, in what way, when, how often and where. This should be agreed and recorded at interview, but also reinforced each time they turn up. The volunteer who is assisting over the long term should also be provided with regular opportunities for supervision in the same way as employed members of the staff team.

Good volunteers with a special contribution to make can be worth their weight in gold. Volunteers who are more concerned with their own needs than those of the client group can be an expensive drain on resources. All volunteers are time-consuming; the staff team needs to be clear about whether they have the necessary resources to expend, and how far channelling resources in this direction will ultimately benefit the client.

6.4 Clients

Clients are rarely seen as a resource, but they should be. One of the greater deprivations of the increasing frailty of old age is the diminishing opportunity to give to others, either in tangible ways or in service. Good practice looks for ways to make good that deficit by recognising and utilising retained abilities, whether it is to ask Arthur to wash up the coffee things to assist busy staff, to ask Vera to help Connie button her cardigan, or to accept Mrs Clark's offer of a knitted dishcloth. The greater the range of retained abilities, the greater the opportunity for a client to make a contribution.

6.5 Equipment and budgets

6.5.1 Budgets for equipment and materials

All care settings should have a budget specifically designated for activity provision. It is unacceptable to expect that activity provision will be self-financing (where the budget is determined by what clients and staff can make and then sell) as it is in some care settings. Such a practice severely constrains the kind of activities that may be provided and determines that activity staff are task-led and money-led, rather than needs-led. This is not to say that clients shouldn't contribute to the budget through things that they can make and sell. This should be encouraged if it is the client's positive choice, but it should never be the sole source of funding for activities.

It is not possible in a book such as this to indicate what a satisfactory budget should be. The size of the budget will depend upon the size and nature of the unit, and upon the unit's commitment to activity provision. The larger the better, but a lot can be done with even a relatively small budget through the use of equipment loans and 'do-it-yourself' (see 6.5.3).

Ideally a budget relating to activity provision should be administered by the activity coordinator and a senior manager. There should be some consultation and corporate decision-making about exactly how much is spent and on what. If there is no activity coordinator, a senior manager should take responsibility in consultation with the activity organiser.

6.5.2 Equipment and materials

As with budgets, it is not possible for a book of this nature to specify what makes a good stock of equipment and materials; this will depend upon the client group. But for the practitioner who is building up a stock from scratch, or trying to identify deficits within existing stock, the rule of thumb is to ask oneself whether there is a range of equipment to meet a range of needs such as those listed below.

- *Self-care*. Hair and manicure equipment, make-up, toiletries, shoe cleaning items, mending kits, etc.
- *Creativity*. Music, musical instruments, karaoke, art, collage and modelling materials, cooking materials, horticultural items, craft materials.
- *Cognitive*. Books, magazines, newspapers, card games, table games, word and number games, jigsaws, quizzes, reminiscence materials, typewriter, computer.
- *Physical exercise*. Balls, balloons, scarves, parachute, skittles, bowls, croquet, target games, suitable music.
- *Sensory*. Rummage bag, feely bag, smell box, textured games, perfumes, massage creams, lava lamps, fibre optics.
- *Sensory impairment*. There is now a huge range of self-care and leisure equipment on the market for people who are visually or hearing

impaired. Catalogues are available from the RNIB and RNID (see Appendix 4: Addresses).

- *Daily living*. Equipment for making drinks and snacks, for doing a hand wash and ironing, for washing and wiping up, for tending plants and flowers, for cleaning and dusting.

6.5.3 Equipment and materials on the cheap

Items purchased from catalogues tend to be extremely expensive. The wise activity provider will give a little time to investigating alternative sources. There are two main sources of inexpensive materials and equipment. The first is to make them yourself. For example, a 'smell box' from the catalogue can cost upwards of £50, but can be made quickly and easily for a pound or two. The second is to investigate equipment loans. Many libraries and museums now operate loan schemes for reminiscence artefacts; some organisations hold a large and varied stock of equipment that can be borrowed by individual units.

Other options are to keep an eye on junk shops (good source of reminiscence items), jumble sales (good source of reminiscence and sensory items), gadget shops (good source of inexpensive sensory items), markets in holiday countries (good source of all kinds of things). It is also worth cultivating relationships with shops and factories for anything they might otherwise throw away, such as plants and flowers, offcuts of fabric, paper and card. Activity providers do tend to become inveterate collectors.

6.5.4 Monitoring equipment and materials

It is sadly true to say that equipment for activity provision has a distinct tendency to 'walk' or to get damaged or lost and the activity provider needs to try and keep tabs on it. There is a certain inevitability about this, particularly when a large number of staff are using items. A lockable store cupboard is essential for times when items are not in use, but this must always be accessible for any staff wishing to use an item with a client. Keys need to be held centrally and not just by the activity provider.

6.6 Community resources

6.6.1 Establishing a database

Every care setting should have (or work towards establishing) a database of local community and national resources which can be tapped for specialist contributions to activity provision. Such a database takes time to build up and the task should not fall just to the activity provider. Anybody with a specialist knowledge of local amenities, or of national groups and organisations can provide information and contact details. Care settings within a locality can assist one another in this by sharing information.

The database is probably best kept in a small card file to make it easily acceptable to all staff, but it can of course be held on computer provided that most people can access it without difficulty.

6.6.2 The resources

The kinds of resources the activity provider needs to know about include:

- Libraries and library services
- Museums
- Churches and their outreach services and projects
- Schools and colleges (particularly any intergenerational projects)
- Elder care organisations
- Service veterans organisations
- Arts organisations
- Disability organisations
- Ethnic organisations
- Complementary therapies
- Entertainers

- Easy access transport
- Easy access shopping
- Pubs and restaurants
- Theatres and cinemas
- Swimming and sports facilities.

6.7 Building resources – internal facilities

Any care setting is, of course, constrained by the bricks and mortar that give it its shape. Some buildings are purpose-built, some are not. Some are well-designed, some are not. Staff teams have to make the best of their building's basic frame. The design of residential settings for frail older people is a specialist matter ripe for urgent research and development. This document can only recommend general ideals.

6.7.1 Activity areas

The care setting should have a range of different rooms or areas in which activities can take place. It is true that some activities can take place in a main lounge setting, but this is not always appropriate. The ideal setting would have large and small areas for group activities and for the privacy of one-to-one interaction. Some areas should be conducive to comfort and relaxation, and some to activity and work. An area with an uncarpeted floor is useful, where a mess can freely be made with art or gardening materials.

Space is critically important for ease of access and mobility. Appropriate seating is important for the same reason, and also for the purposes of facilitating different activities. Clients should be able to sit in easy chairs for discussion or listening to music, but have the option to transfer to upright chairs for exercise or for working at a table. Chairs of different heights and widths are also important.

6.7.2 Decor and lighting

Decor is a matter of taste of course, and clients in residential settings should have the facility to decorate their own room where possible. Communal areas should be in light colours, with bolder colours indicating significant areas such as toilets. Pictorial and written direction and door signs are an important aid where people may have mental health impairments. Creative staff and clients in some care settings have 'personalised' and brightened boring decor with murals and collage, with clients' art work and with themed artefacts relating to local history or reminiscence.

Lighting generally needs to be central and diffuse. Small table lamps may look cosy and homely, but they are fairly useless for the purpose of clear vision. Portable anglepoise lamps or spotlighting is very helpful for those wanting to engage in close work.

6.7.3 Kitchens

For most older people whose formative years were spent in a family context, the kitchen was the hub of the home. It was where mother was, where everyday chores were, where meals were taken, and often (in the pre-central heating era), where it was warmest. Kitchens retain a significant place in many people's memory and affections, and they have a great importance in activity provision.

They are the place of long-familiar activities hard-wired into the memory, they encourage a 'family' intimacy in small groups and they are associated with the pleasure of eating and drinking together. Care settings need to have well-supervised kitchen areas where people can make drinks and snacks, have a coffee and a chat, and gather round to stir the Christmas pudding or organise the party food.

6.8 Building resources – external facilities

As with the building, the garden and exterior facilities of a unit are 'givens' and there is not always much we can do to alter the basic size and shape. Content is a little easier to vary if finances are available.

6.8.1 Basic requirements

Any unit should have an area of lawn and flowerbeds, walkways leading to points of interest and plenty of comfortable and sheltered seating. A greenhouse is a real bonus for encouraging clients in gardening tasks.

6.8.2 Requirements for physical disability

Safe access is a priority. Walkways should be wide enough to accommodate wheelchairs, with solid and level surfaces and handrails for their full length. Depending upon the size of the area, seating should be available at regular intervals. Raised flowerbeds enable clients to garden from a standing position without bending, or from a seated position. Long-handled garden tools are a useful accessory to the raised bed.

6.8.3 Requirements for dementia

The exterior needs to have a secure perimeter unless the unit has a facility for the constant monitoring of clients' whereabouts. A garden can be a rich resource of sensory stimulation; this should be a consideration where the unit has any number of people with a more advanced dementia. Flowers with bold colours and strong scents are important. Herb gardens can add another range of scents, in addition to being useful in the kitchen. Growing fruit and vegetables offers a range of simple and repetitive tasks with a multisensory focus. Wind chimes and water features can add an auditory as well as visual stimulus.

NB: Flowers and plants are occasionally eaten by some people with dementia. Dementia carers should therefore be careful to eliminate any potentially toxic plants from the surroundings. An organisation called Thrive (see Appendix 4: Addresses) can advise.

Chapter 7

Education and Staff Development

7.1 Accredited training

7.1.1 City & Guilds 6977 – Certificate in Providing Therapeutic Activities for Older People

This is an award which has been developed by NAPA in collaboration with City & Guilds. It is a Vocational Award which has been written to a standard similar to NVQ Level 3. It is designed to offer a qualification to the person holding the role of activity coordinator/therapist as understood by this book (see 6.1). City & Guilds recommends that training courses leading to the award allocate 300 hours for teaching and a further 150 hours for practical experience in the workplace. There are five units, as follows:

- Human ageing in health and illness
- Interpersonal communication
- The effective use of resources
- Activities: a therapeutic resource
- Delivering therapeutic activities.

At the time of going to press we are aware of no other accredited award for activity providers. Discussions are currently taking place as to the feasibility of developing an award pitched at Level 2.

7.2 Other training

7.2.1 NAPA short courses

NAPA offers short one- and two-day courses on a range of subjects related to activity provision for older people. At the time of publication, these include:

- Providing effective activity programmes in a care home setting
- Art and craft and creativity
- Special exercise for special people
- Creative writing and emotional healing in dementia
- Using drama with older people
- Life story work with older people
- More to life than a talking book
- Therapeutic activities in dementia care
- Assessment and evaluation in dementia
- Understanding confused and challenging behaviour in dementia.

Further details are available from NAPA.

7.2.2 Other organisations offering short courses

There are many short courses available through other organisations for people who are involved in activity programmes for older people or people with disabilities. See Appendix 4: Addresses for the organisations listed below:

- Age Concern – provides a range of courses on matters relating to the care of older people

- British Association for Services to the Elderly – provides a range of courses on matters relating to the care of older people
- Age Exchange Reminiscence Centre – provides courses on matters relating to using reminiscence with older people
- EXTEND – courses on music with movement for older people and people with disabilities
- Jabadao – courses on using movement as a means of enhancing communication with older people and people with disabilities
- Thrive – courses on horticultural therapy for people with disabilities
- Dementia Training and Consultancy Services – courses and consultancy on matters relating to dementia care.

7.2.3 The Successful Activity Coordinator Training Pack

This is a self-directed learning pack developed by two occupational therapists who are NAPA associates. It is published by Age Concern England and available either from Age Concern England or from NAPA. The pack is in a 'user-friendly' format and takes the student through a series of learning tasks across 11 units. The units are as follows:

- Setting the scene: old age, care homes and occupation
- The effects of ageing and common conditions affecting older people
- The role of the activity coordinator
- Effective communication
- Designing innovative programmes
- Successful group work
- The use of themes
- Therapeutic approaches
- Activities
- Activity and dementia
- Ensuring success.

7.3 Learning by networking

7.3.1 Personal networking

One of the best ways of extending knowledge, solving difficulties and obtaining support in the area of activity provision is to make links with others who are working in the same field. More often than not, activity providers have to take responsibility for their own personal development in this matter, and should endeavour to build for themselves a network of other activity providers and related professionals to whom they can turn for advice and support.

Where possible, activity providers should arrange to visit and spend time with one another in their respective care settings. Where possible within organisations, new activity providers should have an opportunity to work alongside experienced practitioners. The benefits of making connections and building relationships of this kind cannot be underestimated. For the activity provider's own job satisfaction and personal development (and ultimately the client's quality of life), it is vital to avoid isolation. Isolation generally leads to rapid burn-out and the vacating of posts.

7.3.2 NAPA networking

- NAPA sharing days are thrice-yearly networking and training events designed to help activity providers to explore activity-related issues with others from similar care settings.
- A number of NAPA regional groups have been established in different localities across the UK. In every case they are a collective of activity providers and related professionals who have come together for the precise purpose of mutual support and learning. NAPA groups operate relatively autonomously, but are required to maintain strong links with the central committee and to develop within the ethos of NAPA principles and practices.

Further details on the above initiatives can be obtained from NAPA.

7.4 Reflective practice

Reflective practice should be an essential part of the activity provider's working day. The practitioner who does not know how to evaluate his or her interventions and to engage in self-appraisal is a potential health risk for clients.

7.4.1 The nature of reflective practice

Reflective practice is in part intuitive and in part learned. A simple model has been proposed (Fish *et al*, 1991) for those who do not know how to go about it. Practitioners need to put themselves through a four-stage enquiry:

- The facts – consider what actually happened, pinpoint any critical incidents and note what you thought, felt and did at the time
- The review – review the event(s), seeking patterns and meanings and evaluating processes, outcomes and personal views
- The hidden agenda – explore the assumptions, beliefs, customs, attitudes or values that underlie the event(s)
- The connection – consider the implications for practice: what was learned, what assumptions were challenged, what could be changed.

7.4.2 The operation of reflective practice

Reflection should be an integral part of everyday practice. At the end of each day, session or activity, practitioners need to pause momentarily to review and to ask their questions.

Reflection can be carried out alone, but is enriched and extended in the presence of others who can contribute alternative views. Relevant others might be the practitioner's supervisor, other participants in the event(s), or even a disinterested outsider who can bring an objective view.

Time for reflective practice should be built into the practitioner's daily routine as a matter of course. Building opportunities into the timetable requires a little planning and self-discipline initially, but gradually becomes second nature as a routine is established.

7.5 Supervision

7.5.1 The supervisor

The supervisor should preferably be a person somewhat senior to the practitioner who can act as advisor and guide. A senior manager or colleague will be the most likely person. If the unit has contact with an occupational therapist experienced in elder care settings this can be a considerable added bonus – not to replace but to complement the senior unit person. Some form of dual supervision would be ideal.

For the activity coordinator who is already in a management position, peer supervision can be effective. In such a case, the practitioner would seek out an experienced colleague of similar seniority.

7.5.2 The purpose

The purpose of supervision is the personal development of the activity provider in the context of his or her work.

7.5.3 The supervision session

Effective supervision sessions should:

- Be planned and timetabled well in advance
- Be frequent and regular, preferably once every month and at least once every six weeks: new staff may require more frequent supervision
- Be of approximately an hour's duration
- Be structured and led by the supervisor, not by the practitioner
- Review progress since the last meeting
- Clarify the work currently being undertaken
- Identify any current problems and establish how these may be overcome

- Set goals to be achieved by the next meeting
- Be documented, indicating the nature of the discussion and the work undertaken.

CHAPTER 8

Obtaining Specialist Help

8.1 Occupational therapy

8.1.1 The role of the occupational therapist

The occupational therapist is a practitioner who is concerned with any dysfunction in or disruption to a person's occupations of daily living, and who works with the person in manipulating those occupations towards restoring function and/or well-being. Occupational therapists tend to work in specialist areas: some work with physical disability, some work in mental health, some work in the field of learning disability. Though occupational therapists have a common base in using occupations as therapy, the nature of their practice varies considerably between client groups.

8.1.2 What you can ask the occupational therapist for

Very few occupational therapists work in, or have contact with, continuing care settings for older people. And although it might be surprising, very few are experienced in providing therapeutic activities in such settings. They do exist, but they are very thin on the ground and you may have difficulty finding one.

However, most occupational therapists will assist with daily living advice and strategies for independence. Some specialise in advising on, and arranging equipment for, people who have a physical disability.

8.1.3 Making a referral

Most social services departments operate an open referral system, which accepts referrals from any person, lay or professional. It is simply a matter of visiting or telephoning the department headquarters and registering the person's need.

8.2 Physiotherapy

8.2.1 The role of the physiotherapist

The physiotherapist is a practitioner who uses physical therapies such as exercise, manipulation, heat and light in the remediation of impairment and disability. Physiotherapists are trained extensively in anatomy and physiology and kinesiology (the study of movement), and are found working predominantly with people who have mobility problems and movement disorders.

8.2.2 What you can ask a physiotherapist for

The physiotherapist might be consulted regarding any person considered to have difficulties with walking, sitting or standing, on appropriate exercise regimes for the mobility and general fitness of clients, and on problems relating to seating, positioning or handling of the more disabled client.

8.2.3 Making a referral

Services vary across the country, but it would be generally true to say that physiotherapists will only accept referrals through a medical practitioner. A person's own general practice (or general practitioner) will advise.

8.3 Speech and language therapy

8.3.1 The role of the speech and language therapist

The speech and language therapist (SLT) works with people of all ages and with a wide range of communication problems. Some are trained to assess and advise on swallowing difficulties. An integral part of the SLT's role is advising families and carers on how to facilitate communication and this is often the most usual intervention with older people.

8.3.2 What you can ask a speech and language therapist for

Older people are usually referred to the SLT if they are experiencing difficulty with speech, understanding and/or swallowing following a stroke, or if they have a progressive condition such as Parkinson's disease. SLTs can also assess people when it is uncertain if their speech difficulties are due to a dementia or a stroke, and are usually pleased to advise on facilitating communication with all client groups.

8.3.3 Making a referral

SLT services may differ across localities with regard to referral mechanisms. In most areas an open referral system operates, and you can refer a client directly to the local SLT department. If the client needs a swallowing assessment, a written referral signed by a doctor is required. It is always best to refer clients early.

8.4 Services for visual and hearing impairment

By far the best source of information and advice on services for people with visual or hearing impairments are the Royal National Institute for the Blind (RNIB) and the Royal National Institute for the Deaf (RNID). Both organisations offer copious quantities of free literature on all matters relating to their specialist area, will advise over the phone, and can direct the enquirer to sources of assistance within their own locality. See Appendix 4: Addresses.

APPENDIX 1

Sample Categories for Gathering Biographical Data

- Significant life events
- Significant events of the year
- Significant people
- Food and drink preferences
- Preferred style and size of clothing
- Preferred routines and practices for bathing
- Preferred routines and practices for rising/going to bed
- Preferences in self-care routines, such as hairdressing and manicure
- Special needs in communication
- Spirituality and religious practices
- Preferences in relation to music, television, radio, books, newspapers, entertainments
- School, family, friends and pastimes of early years
- Family, friends and pastimes of adult years
- Education, qualifications, National Service and work in adult years
- Family, friends and retirement in later years.

Appendix 2

An Overview of the Literature

The publications cited below are set out as an overview. The reader wishing to consult the original documents can obtain full details from the reference list.

Evidence for the link between activity and health

Havighurst, 1968. There is a positive relationship between social activity and life satisfaction across the life spectrum.

Glass *et al*, 1999. Social and productive activities lower the risk of mortality as much as physical fitness activities and may confer survival benefits.

Csikszentmihalyi, 1975, 1988, 1992. When the challenges of activity are high and personal skills are used to the utmost, we experience an optimum level of well-being.

Rosenzweig *et al*, 1972/Diamond, 1976. The experience of living in an environment enriched with opportunities for activity increases the weight and thickness of the cerebral cortex in experimental rats.

Evidence for the link between inactivity and ill health

Csikszentmihalyi, 1975. Disengagement from the non-instrumental activities of daily living is experienced as deeply distressing and debilitating.

Whiteford, 2000. Occupational deprivation will be experienced by increasing numbers of people globally over the coming millennium.

Bexton *et al,* **1954.** Cognitive and emotional disruption is experienced as a result of deprivation of sensory stimulation.

Corcoran, 1991. The health hazards of bed rest and inactivity.

Asher, 1947. Too much time in bed is dangerous – all systems are negatively affected.

Ryback *et al,* **1971.** The negative effects of prolonged bed rest on young healthy volunteers.

Gravelle, 1985. The effects on health and survival of occupational deprivation through unemployment.

Smith, 1987. The effects on health and survival of occupational deprivation through unemployment.

Robb, 1967. The effects of occupational deprivation and deprivation of all kinds in continuing care settings.

Perrin, 1997c. The low levels of well-being associated with occupational deprivation in continuing care settings for people with dementia.

Cohen & Taylor, 1974. The effects of occupational deprivation in long-term imprisonment.

Keenan, 1992. The effects of occupational deprivation in long-term imprisonment.

Armstrong-Esther *et al,* **1994.** The failure of nurses to engage older patients in activities and interactions.

Nolan *et al,* **1995.** The failure of nurses to engage older patients in activities and interactions.

Evidence for the link between activity and health in elder care settings

Crump, 1991. The provision of activity is a basic right of the older person in a care setting; the absence of meaningful activity could be interpreted as abuse.

Powell *et al*, 1979. An indoor gardening activity significantly improves sustained engagement in a residential home.

Jenkins *et al*, 1977. Recreational materials significantly improve sustained engagement in a residential home.

Pratt, 1987. The positive effects of engaging an older person in activity – a case study.

Bower, 1967. Functional, cognitive and emotional improvements in the context of a sustained programme of occupational, sensory and environmental stimulation in a continuing care setting.

Perrin, 1997b. The effects of appropriate occupation upon the well-being of people with dementia.

Appendix 3

Care Homes for Older People: National Minimum Standards

Standard 3 – Needs Assessment

3.1 New service users are admitted only on the basis of a full assessment undertaken by people trained to do so, and to which the prospective service user, his/her representatives (if any) and relevant professionals have been party.

3.2 For individuals referred through care management arrangements, the registered person obtains a summary of the care management (health and social services) assessment and a copy of the care plan produced for care management purposes.

3.3 For individuals, who are self-funding and without a care management assessment/care plan, the registered person carries out a needs assessment covering:

- Personal care and physical well-being
- Diet and weight, including dietary preferences

- Sight, hearing and communication
- Oral health
- Foot care
- Mobility and dexterity
- History of falls
- Continence
- Medical usage
- Mental state and cognition
- Social interests, hobbies, religious and cultural needs
- Personal safety and risk
- Carer and family involvement and other social contacts/relationships

3.4 Each service user has a plan of care for daily living, and longer term outcomes, based on the care management assessment and care plan or on the home's own needs assessment.

3.5 The registered nursing input required by service users in homes which provide nursing care is determined by NHS registered nurses using a recognised assessment tool, according to Department of Health guidelines.

APPENDIX 4

Addresses

Age Concern National Training Office

89 Station Road   Tel 0191 266 7488

Forest Hall

Newcastle-upon-Tyne

NE12 8AQ

Age Exchange Reminiscence Centre

11 Blackheath Village   Tel 0208 318 9105

London

SE3 9LA

British Association for Services to the Elderly (BASE)

119 Hassell Street   Tel 01483 451036

Newcastle-under-Lyme

ST5 1AX

City & Guilds
1 Giltspur Street   Tel 0207 294 2468
London
EC1A 9DD

Dementia Training and Consultancy Services
TLC Care Services   Tel 0207 749 2396
St Leonards   or 0207 729 6335
Nuttall Street
London
N1 5LZ

EXTEND (recreational movement to music)
22 Maltings Drive   Tel 01582 832760
Wheathampstead
Herts
AL4 8JQ

NAPA
Unit 5.12, 5th Floor   Tel 0207 831 3320
Bondway Commercial Centre
71 Bondway
London
SW8 1SQ

National Centre for Movement, Learning and Health (Jabadao)
The Yard   Tel 0113 236 3311
Viaduct Street
Stanningley
Leeds
LS28 6AU

Royal National Institute for the Blind (RNIB)

224 Great Portland Street   Tel 0345 66 99 99
London
W1N 6AA

Royal National Institute for the Deaf (RNID)

PO Box 16464   Tel 0870 605 0123
London
EC1Y 8TT

Thrive (horticultural therapy for people with disabilities)

The Geoffrey Udall Building   Tel 0118 988 5688
Trunkwell Park
Beech Hill
Reading
RG7 2AT

References

Armstrong-Esther C, Browne K & McAfee J, 1994, 'Elderly patients: still clean and sitting quietly', *Journal of Advanced Nursing* 19, pp264–71.

Asher R, 1947, 'The dangers of going to bed', *British Medical Journal* 2, p967.

Barton R, 1959, *Institutional Neurosis*, Wright, Bristol.

Bexton W, Heron W *et al*, 1954, 'Effects of decreased variation in the sensory environment', *Canadian Journal of Psychology* 8(2), pp70–76.

Bower H, 1967, 'Sensory stimulation and the treatment of senile dementia', *Medical Journal of Australia* 1(22), pp1113–19.

Bruce E, 2000, 'Looking after well-being: a tool for evaluation', *Journal of Dementia Care* 8(6), pp25–27.

Cohen S & Taylor L, 1974, *Psychological Survival: The Experience of Long-Term Imprisonment*, Vintage, New York.

Corocoran P, 1991, 'Use it or lose it: the hazards of bed rest and inactivity', *The Western Journal of Medicine* 154(5), pp536–38.

Crump A, 1991, 'Promoting self-esteem', *Nursing the Elderly* March/April, pp19–21.

Csikszentmihalyi M, 1975, *Beyond Boredom and Anxiety*, Jossey-Bass, California.

Csikszentmihalyi M & Csikszentmihalyi I, 1988, *Optimal Experience: Psychological Studies of Flow in Consciousness*, Cambridge University Press, Cambridge.

Csikszentmihalyi M, 1992, *Flow: The Psychology of Happiness*, Rider, London.

Diamond M, 1976, 'Anatomical brain changes produced by environment', McGaugh J & Petrinovich L (eds), *Knowing, Thinking and Believing*, Plenum Press, New York.

Fish D, Twinn & Purr, 1991, *Promoting Reflection*, West London Institute of Higher Education, London.

Glass T, Mendes de Leon C et al, 1999, 'Population-based study of social and productive activities as predictors of survival among elderly Americans', *British Medical Journal* 319, pp478–83.

Gravelle H, 1985, *Does Unemployment Kill?*, Nuffield Provincial Hospitals Trust, London.

Havighurst R, 1968, 'Personality and patterns of ageing', *Gerontologist* 8, pp20–3.

Jenkins J, Felce D et al, 1977, 'Increasing engagement in activity of residents in old people's homes by providing recreational materials', *Behaviour Research and Therapy* 15, pp429–34.

Keenan B, 1992, *An Evil Cradling*, Vintage, London.

Morris D, 1964, 'The response of animals to a restricted environment', *Symposium of the Zoological Society of London* 13, pp99–118.

Mulhall D, (forthcoming), *The Functional Performance Record* (details available from NAPA).

Nolan M, Grant G & Nolan J, 1995, 'Busy doing nothing: activity and interaction levels amongst differing populations of elderly patients', *Journal of Advanced Nursing* 22, pp528–38.

Perrin T, 1997a, 'Occupational need in dementia care: a literature review and implications for practice', *Healthcare in Later Life* 2(3), pp166–76.

Perrin T, 1997b, 'The role and value of occupation in severe dementia', Unpublished PhD thesis, University of Bradford.

Perrin T, 1997c, 'Occupational need in severe dementia: a descriptive study', *Journal of Advanced Nursing* 25, pp934–41.

Powell L, Felce D *et al*, 1979, 'Increasing engagement in a home for the elderly by providing an indoor gardening activity', *Behaviour Research and Therapy* 17, pp127–35.

Pratt M, 1987, 'When health means afternoon tea', *Kentucky Nurse* Nov/Dec, p16.

Robb B, 1967, *Sans Everything: A Case to Answer*, Nelson, London.

Rosenzweig M, Bennett E & Diamond M, 1972, 'Brain changes in response to experience', *Scientific American* 2(226), pp22–29.

Ryback R, Trimble T *et al*, 1971, 'Psychobiologic effects of prolonged weightlessness – bedrest – of young healthy volunteers', *Aerospace Medicine* 42, pp408–15.

Smith R, 1987, *Unemployment and Health: A Disaster and A Challenge*, Oxford University Press, Oxford.

Whiteford G, 2000, 'Occupational deprivation: global challenge for the new millennium', *British Journal of Occupational Therapy* 63(5), pp200–4.